IDA JEAN ORLANDO

Notes on Nursing Theories

SERIES EDITORS

Chris Metzger McQuiston
Doctoral Candidate, Wayne State University

Adele A. Webb
College of Nursing, University of Akron

Notes on Nursing Theories is a series of monographs designed to provide the reader with a concise description of conceptual frameworks and theories in nursing. Each monograph includes a biographical sketch of the theorist, origin of the theory, assumptions, concepts, propositions, examples for application to practice and research, a glossary of terms, and a bibliography of classic works, critiques, and research.

IDA JEAN ORLANDO

A Nursing Process Theory

Norma Jean Schmieding

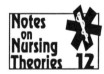
Notes
on
Nursing
Theories 12

SAGE Publications
International Educational and Professional Publisher
Newbury Park   London   New Delhi

For information address:

SAGE Publications, Inc.
2455 Teller Road
Newbury Park, California 91320

SAGE Publications Ltd.
6 Bonhill Street
London EC2A 4PU
United Kingdom

SAGE Publications India Pvt. Ltd.
M-32 Market
Greater Kailash I
New Delhi 110 048 India

Printed in the United States of America

Library of Congress Cataloging-in-Publication Data

Schmiedling, Norma Jean.
    Ida Jean Orlando: a nursing process theory / Norma Jean Schmiedling.
        p. cm. — (Notes on nursing theories; v. 12)
    Includes bibliographical references.
    ISBN 0-8039-4907-3 (cl). — ISBN 0-8039-4908-1 (pbk.)
    1. Nurse and patient. 2. Nursing—Philosophy. 3. Orlando, Ida Jean. I. Title. II. Series.
    [DNLM: 1. Orlando, Ida Jean. 2. Nursing Process. 3. Nursing Theory. WY 100 S3541 1993]
RT86.3.S52 1993
610.73'01—dc20
DNLM/DLC   93-5729

93 94 95 96   10 9 8 7 6 5 4 3 2 1

Sage Production Editor: Diane S. Foster

Contents

Foreword

A major value of nursing theory is its utility in helping nurses distinguish actions that form the core of professional nursing practice from actions that are the responsibility of other health-care providers. At the time that Orlando's theory was evolving, much of nursing care practice involved assisting physicians so more effective medical care could be provided to patients. Nursing science was in the embryonic phase and practices were based on medically derived principles or on anecdotal data. Comparatively few nurses questioned this approach and many perceived their professional obligations to patients as secondary to their medical assistant responsibilities.

Orlando had the wisdom to question the prevailing mode of thinking about nursing practice. She recognized that nursing could not be a profession unless it had a distinct function or goal. Without the articulation of that goal, she knew that nurses would continue to function as paraprofessionals to medicine and would never develop a science of nursing. Orlando's inductive studies revealed that outcomes improved when the nurse was *patient* centered. Her data enabled her to define the nurse's professional responsibility and to delineate the process for fulfilling that obligation. This monograph provides an excellent description and analysis of that important work.

The author, Dr. Norma Jean Schmieding, is eminently qualified to present this theory. As a young nurse Dr. Schmieding found herself questioning many aspects of the nurse's role. She wondered about all of the activities that consumed nurses' time without benefiting patients. She knew the value of nursing to patients was being diluted by these routines. She recognized that tasks rather than patients often preoccupied nurses, and yet was not sure how to change all of this. Then she encountered Ida Jean Orlando, who was teaching deliberative nursing process at McLean Hospital in Massachusetts. Her response was relief. Her concerns about nursing practice and her belief in the salience of the discipline to patients were validated.

Dr. Schmieding used the process she learned from Orlando in her own practice. Later, upon assuming the role of director of nursing, she used the theory to guide practice within the nursing service she administered. This helped other nurses to identify their professional role, and the quality of nursing care improved greatly. While a doctoral student and recently, Schmieding has authored numerous articles based on the theory. In fact, Orlando's work was the focus of her doctoral dissertation.

This monograph provides the reader with an understanding of Orlando's work from the perspective of an individual who has practiced, studied, and taught it. The theory has laid a foundation for nursing practice and nursing science. Dr. Schmieding has presented it with skill and precision.

LOIS A. HAGGERTY, PhD, RN
Associate Professor
Boston College
School of Nursing

Preface

Nursing, as a noble profession, occurs through a process that involves the nurse and the individual in need of the nurse's help. When a nurse and a patient first meet neither has much information about the other. Nurses never know in advance what reaction they will have toward the patient nor the patient's reaction toward them. Nonetheless, what transpires in this contact has implications for the patient's welfare as well as the nurse's fulfillment of her or his professional responsibility and work satisfaction. Because the majority of practice occurs in face-to-face contact, nurses need skills to discover the meaning of the situation.

Each nursing theory provides a different view of nursing that is intended to help the nurse to nurse. The focus may be the patient, the nurse, or the nurse-patient process. Orlando's theory focuses on the nurse-patient process and helps the nurse understand what happens, how it happens, and its relationship to the process of helping the patient. The patient is an active participant in this process.

Although this book is intended for undergraduate students, it can serve as a review for graduate students as well as for nurses in health-care organizations who are searching for a useful nursing practice theory. It is not a critique of Orlando's theory but rather a distillation of the theory's major components. The sections on propositions, research, and clinical application are intended to convey the relevance of Orlando's theory to practice as well as to pose areas for further research. The literature references provide sources for those who wish to explore further the theory and related works.

To understand a theory one must study it and experiment with its application to practice. Only in this way can nurses select a theory most helpful to their practice. I hope students will find Orlando's theory useful. The beauty of Orlando's theory is that it does not preclude the use of other theories and concepts, including nursing theories. Rather they are resources from which the nurse can draw to help the patient.

For years I have studied and used Orlando's theory in practice, teaching, research, and administration and can attest to its usefulness. Each time I delve into Orlando's theory I am amazed by its clarity and the simplicity with which she describes the theory. I hope the readers of this book will find the theory as compelling as I have.

Biographical Sketch of the Nurse Theorist:
Ida Jean Orlando, BS, MA, RN

Born: August 12, 1926
Diploma: New York Medical College, Lower Fifth Avenue
    Hospital, School of Nursing, New York
BS: St. John's University, Brooklyn, NY
MA: Teachers College, Columbia University, New York
Previous Positions: Associate Professor of Nursing and
    Director of the Graduate Program in Mental Health
    Psychiatric Nursing, Yale School of Nursing, New Haven,
    CT; Clinical Nursing Consultant, McLean Hospital,
    Belmont, MA, and Director, Research Project: Two
    Systems of Nursing in a Psychiatric Hospital; Assistant
    Director of Nursing for Education and Research,
    Metropolitan State Hospital, Waltham, MA; National and
    international consultant and speaker

1

Origin of the Theory

Orlando formulated her nursing process theory in the late 1950s while principal investigator of the Yale School of Nursing Project. This project, funded by a National Institute of Mental Health Grant, was entitled "Integration of Mental Health Principles in the Basic Nursing Curriculum." The grant's purpose was to identify factors inhibiting and enhancing the integration of mental health concepts in the nursing curriculum. To establish these factors, principles guiding effective nursing practice had to be identified. Orlando's book *The Dynamic Nurse-Patient Relationship,*[1,2] published in 1961, was an outcome of this project and has been highly acclaimed for its influence on nursing education and practice. According to Orlando (1961), the book's content was to contribute to concerns about (a) the nurse-patient relationship, (b) the nurse's professional role and identity, and (c) knowledge development distinct to nursing. Orlando's theory radically shifted the nurse's focus from the medical diagnosis and automatic activities, decided upon without patient participation, to the patient's immediate experience and whether the patient was helped by the nurse's action. Orlando was, and remains, one of a few nurse theorists who explicitly include active patient participation as integral to their theory. Orlando's formulations are integrated into much of current education and practice literature, often unintentionally, without recognition of the source. Orlando's theory has become a part of many nurses' thinking and practice.

Following her initial work at Yale, Orlando further refined her theory through a National Institute of Mental Health Public Health Service research grant while she was a clinical nurse consultant at McLean Hospital, Belmont, Massachusetts. In this grant Orlando assessed the relevance of her previous formulations, trained and evaluated nurses in the use of these formulations, and tested the validity of her formulations. Her second book, *The Discipline and Teaching of Nursing Process,* published in 1972, contained the study's research results and the extended formulations of her theory, which included a definition of the entire nursing practice system.

It is important to place in a historical context the critical nursing issues at the time of a theory's development. In the 1950s nursing was struggling to define its work and to move nursing education into the mainstream of higher education and away from apprentice models of learning. In nursing schools there was a move to incorporate new knowledge, such as psychiatric principles, into nursing curricula and to move away from the medical model as the basis of nursing education.

These issues are reflected in Orlando's thinking (1961). For example, she writes that principles and concepts from other fields enable nurses to explain their observations of patients, and the activities that are carried out in relation to these observations. However, she cautions that these principles are derived from the study of particular aspects of the behaving human organism and not from nursing practice. Orlando (1961) recognizes the importance of making this distinction because general principles, which explain behavior or promote health, remain valid even when the immediate and individual nature of the nursing situation is not considered. Nurses, however, have to deal with specific situations to which general knowledge cannot be arbitrarily applied. Nonetheless, Orlando (1961) acknowledges that theories and practices from other fields may be used by nurses as needed; therefore the broader the nurse's knowledge, the greater the resources upon which the nurse may draw when necessary to help the patient. This belief supports incorporating a liberal arts foundation into basic nursing education. Thus, Orlando recognizes the importance of using knowledge developed in other fields while at the same time emphasizing the distinctiveness of the discipline of professional nursing.

Orlando (1972) maintains that nursing problems were associated with the absence of a distinct function of professional nursing, which, in turn, left nurses without a clear concept of what outcome should be achieved with patients. Because professional authority is derived from a distinct professional function, she believed this lack of specificity of function had interfered with the development of a framework to evaluate professional nurses' activities. It also had interfered with the study of the nursing process and the development of the content needed to achieve the outcome of a distinct function (Orlando, 1972).

A practice discipline needs theories to guide the practitioners' actions. Theories unique to nursing are derived from the observation of nursing phenomena. Many nursing theories have been developed from borrowed theories adopted or adapted to nursing. Orlando was one of the earliest nurse theorists, and one of the first to develop a nursing theory inductively from the empirical study of nurses' practice.

The development of scientific knowledge, according to Kuhn, must take into account how that science is actually practiced (Schmieding, 1983). The origin of Orlando's theory emanates from her systematic observations of nursing practice. She was the first nurse to use a participant-observer field methodology approach to theory development. This qualitative methodology more recently has become an accepted approach for knowledge development in nursing.

For years Orlando was preoccupied with the thought that she did not know what a nurse should produce when professionally trained. Her principal investigator position at Yale provided her with a clinical setting to observe the interactions between nurses and patients directly. For 3 years Orlando recorded "only what I heard the person say and what I saw in the sequence in which it took place" (Pelletier, 1976, p. 18).[3] She then examined the content of these 2,000 nurse-patient records and only was able to categorize them into two mutually exclusive sets that she labeled "good nursing" and "bad nursing." Recommendations from psychiatrists and sociologists for a different approach to the data's categorization failed to establish mutually exclusive categories. Orlando then presented a random selection of these records to nurses with dissimilar characteristics and backgrounds. Strikingly, all these nurses agreed with Orlando's categorization of what was judged good and bad nursing. Orlando exclaimed:

And then the light dawned. I decided that if the anecdotal account was the only material available to base the judgment on, then what made good or bad nursing happen had to be contained in the anecdotal record from which all those uniform judgments were made. Stated another way: specific items and/or conditions producing the good or bad outcomes had to be contained in the records which were so judged and could therefore be commonly identified. (Pelletier, 1976, p. 22)

Deliberative formulations were found in the outcomes judged good nursing, whereas in bad nursing the outcomes contained automatic nursing formulations.

In the records judged as good the nurse's focus was on the immediate verbal and nonverbal behavior of the patient from the beginning through the end of the contact; whereas in those judged as bad the nurse's focus was on prescribed activity or something that had nothing to do with the patient's behavior. (Pelletier, 1976, p. 23)

In contacts where good nursing occurred the nurse found out, from the patient's viewpoint, what was happening to the patient and identified the patient's distress. The nurse also determined why the patient was distressed and recognized that the patient was unable to relieve the distress without the nurse's help. This observation led Orlando to "the inescapable conclusion that the function of professional nursing is to find out and meet the patient's immediate needs for HELP" (Pelletier, 1976, p. 24). These findings led Orlando to conclude that the outcome of the professional nurse's work is found in the immediate behavior of the patient and that a professional service had not transpired until the patient's immediate behavior was improved from the patient's point of view.

Orlando does not acknowledge any previous work as the source of her theoretical thinking. Some scholars believe she was influenced by and influenced other nurse theorists. Andrews (1989), Leonard and Crane (1990), and Meleis (1991) note the similarities of her work to that of Peplau (1952) in terms of her focus on interpersonal relationships and the commonality of their definition of nursing. Peplau and Orlando have similarities in that they both view nursing as a dynamic process that includes the patient as an integral part of the problem-solving process and their theories each evolved from their direct work with patients. Despite these similarities, Peplau's thinking was greatly influenced by Harry Stack Sullivan, whereas Orlando's thinking and her theory's content appear to have been more significantly influenced by people with whom she was associated at Teachers College, Columbia University.

During the time while Orlando was enrolled at Teachers College in the master's program for mental health consultation, its dean, Louise McManus, was involved nationally in defining nursing. She wrote about the nature of professional nursing and stressed the uniqueness of each situation and that automatic fixed habits of response were insufficient or inadequate as the basis of nursing practice (McManus, 1948). The uniqueness of each situation and the inadequacy of nursing actions based on automatic fixed responses can be seen in Orlando's formulations. Ruth Gilbert (1940, 1951),[4] who wrote *The Public Health Nurse and Her Patient,* was Orlando's teacher for public health nursing. Gilbert focused attention on the dynamics of behavior and on establishing the nurse-patient relationship. In stressing the benefits of mental hygiene for nursing practice, Gilbert notes that it provides "a deliberate, observant, objective way of working, a habit of stopping to question and to think through what the behavior of the patient may mean in relation to a situation, and how the nurse herself relates to that situation" (1940, p. 1). Some similarities between Gilbert's work and Orlando's can be noted in that both place emphasis on the deliberativeness of the nurse's action and on understanding the dynamics and meaning of a patient's behavior.

L. Thomas Hopkins, another person at Columbia whose work may have influenced Orlando, taught educational courses in which Orlando was enrolled. Orlando specifically identifies him as attracting her attention through his conception of the learning process (personal communication, Orlando, October 25, 1985). The core of Hopkins's (1941, 1954) work centers around the influence of past experiences on the meaning of the present situation and on the importance of perceptions in determining behavior. He stressed that behavior emanates from and is validated in experience. The origin of his work can be traced to Kilpatrick (1925, 1941) who in turn acknowledges John Dewey as having the most formative influence on his work. The similarity to Dewey's (1933, 1938) ideas can be seen in the writings of the three people just cited as well as in Orlando's theory.

Regardless of the origin of Orlando's theory, the centrality of the patient is ever present in her theoretical thinking. She believes that the " 'core of practice' 'should' be what it has been and continues to be—the inability of the individual(s) 'to nurse' the self and the self alone cannot identify or get the needed help" (Pelletier, 1980, p. 8). According to Orlando, professional nursing is required when the cause of the inability to care for the self is not known or clearly understood by the person or the nurse before the nurse's investigation of the situation is conducted (Pelletier, 1980).

Orlando's emphasis on obtaining the patient's perspective and involvement in determining the nurse's activity as well as for evaluating the results of the activity is of central importance to her nursing process theory. Orlando's theory was a major force in shifting the nurse's focus away from assisting the physician to finding out and meeting the patient's immediate needs.

Notes

1. Republished by the National League for Nursing in 1990.

2. When Orlando developed her theory the term *patient* was used; therefore throughout this book *patient* rather than *client* is used. In addition, masculine pronouns were used for patients and feminine for nurses; this is noted in some direct quotes.

3. Pelletier is Orlando's married name.

4. Ruth Gilbert recommended Orlando for her position at Yale University School of Nursing.

2

Assumptions of the Theory

Each nursing theory contains assumptions that are explicit or implied. Assumptions are premises accepted by the theorist as given and true, self-evident, and unquestioned (Barnum, 1990). They "are the taken-for-granted statements of the theory. . . . They may or may not represent the shared beliefs of the discipline" (Meleis, 1991, p. 13). Assumptions are important because "they describe that state of being out of which the nursing theory grows. Underlying assumptions are the starting points of the . . . [theorist's] reasoning" (Barnum, 1990, p. 20). In evaluating a theory's assumptions a nurse should consider whether they reflect the real world of nursing and whether the theory is logically consistent with its assumptions. According to Marriner-Tomey (1989), in order to accept as true the theory about the phenomenon one must accept the assumptions as true.

Orlando developed her theory in the late 1950s before the nursing profession began to study theory development systematically. Therefore, Orlando, like most of the early nurse theorists, did not explicitly identify the theory's concepts, assumptions, and propositions systematically. Nonetheless, her theory contains assumptions about the nursing profession, nurses, patients, and the nature of nurse-patient interaction. The following implied assumptions are presented along with Orlando's thoughts related to them.

Assumptions About Nursing

Assumption 1

Nursing is a distinct profession separate from other disciplines.
Orlando (1987) asserts that nurses are independent professionals by
virtue of their license to practice nursing. Her view that doctor's
orders are for the patient, not the nurse, conveys the thrust of her
conviction of this assumption (Pelletier, 1967). She believes that
nursing's failure to articulate a function distinct from medicine, and
other professions, has kept nursing on a dependent path. As a result,
health administrators, medical authorities, and health policies continue to push nursing down a dependent path that has served non-
nursing interests (Orlando, 1985, 1987). Only a radical independent
path would cause health-care policy makers to consider fully the
importance of professional nursing services (Orlando & Dugan,
1989). This distinction would help nurses, as a collective body, to
develop the independent organization and delivery of services
within the competitive health-care system (Orlando & Dugan, 1989).
A distinct professional function provides the independent authority
and autonomy needed to achieve this distinctiveness.

Assumption 2

Professional nursing has a distinct function and product (outcome).
Nursing's failure to identify a distinct function has thwarted the
development of a theoretical framework upon which to base professional nursing practice and the training of professional nurses
(Orlando, 1972). It also has undermined the profession's ability to
build a coherent knowledge base (Orlando & Dugan, 1989). The
distinct function should characterize every activity of every nurse
while practicing nursing; therefore, it must be identifiable in each
nurse-patient contact (Pelletier, 1976). The function justifies nursing's work as a profession and remains constant regardless of the
patient's age, diagnosis, medical care status, or whether cared for at
home or in an institution or agency (Orlando, 1972). The focus of
professional nursing is the patient's immediate experience. Orlando
(1987) believes nursing might lose its intrinsic character and go

down the dependent path if nursing does not collectively clearly articulate its unique function.

Orlando thinks the lack of a distinct function has inhibited nursing's demonstration of the product (outcome) of that function through practice and research, as well as interfered in the development of the content required to achieve the product of the distinct function (Pelletier, 1976). A distinct product would clarify what form the result would take after the nurse fulfills the function. This distinct product is something the patient cannot produce alone or get from anyone else who is not trained to practice professional nursing (Pelletier, 1976). Implicit in this assumption is that effective practice can be empirically identified.

Assumption 3

There is a difference between lay and professional nursing. Orlando (1983) thinks the nursing profession should provide the public with the distinction between lay and professional nursing. According to Orlando (1961) any person nurses another when she or he carries the burden of responsibility for those things that the person cannot do alone. Orlando and Dugan (1989) write that lay nursing is a transmitted social behavior found in all cultures and includes encouragement, nurturance, nourishment, protection, and curative care. This assistance can be provided to the self or to another by almost anybody. The activity is routine, repetitive, or custodial in nature. When these efforts fail people suffer distress and are helpless because they are unaware of and unable to identify the cause of the distress. "In contrast to 'lay' nursing, professional nursing is required when the 'causes' of the individual's inability 'to nurse' the self (or another as with family members) are NOT known or clearly understood by the individual(s) or the nurse. That is, not known *before* the nurse's professional investigation is conducted" (Pelletier, 1980, pp. 4-5).

A professional nurse identifies both the cause of the distress and the individual help required to relieve the distress, and designs the activity to meet the need for help. The effect of the activity, the alleviation of distress, is noted in the patient's verbal and nonverbal behavior (Orlando & Dugan, 1989). The distinction between lay and professional nursing would clarify nursing's societal responsibility.

Assumption 4

Nursing is aligned with medicine. In Orlando's early work the nurse's access to the patient was through medicine. Although she states that traditionally nursing has been aligned with medicine, Orlando consistently emphasizes the difference in the two professions' responsibility to the patient. Physicians place patients under the nurse's care when patients cannot meet their own needs for help or because they need help in following the prescribed treatment or diagnostic plan (Orlando, 1961). Medicine is responsible for the prevention and treatment of disease, whereas nursing is responsible for offering help to patients for their physical and mental comfort while they are under medical treatment or supervision (Orlando, 1961). In her later writings Orlando clearly states that nursing is practiced wherever a person is in need of its service. This service is provided to people both sick and well, with or without a diagnosed disease, and takes place within or outside institutions (Orlando, 1972, 1987).

Assumptions About Patients

Assumption 1

Patients' needs for help are unique. Because patients are unique the help a nurse provides must be specifically geared to each patient's immediate needs for help (Orlando, 1961). Orlando developed specific guidelines for nurses to use to uncover the meaning of a patient's unique experience.

Assumption 2

Patients have an initial inability to communicate their needs for help. According to Orlando (1961) nurses must realize that patients cannot clearly state the nature and meaning of their distress or need without the nurse's help or without having a previously established helpful relationship (Orlando, 1961). Without this recognition patients' distress will not be identified. Consequently this delay may seriously threaten the patient's condition or exacerbate his or her discomfort (Orlando, 1961). Considering patients' initial inability to communicate clearly, nurses should assume that patients' behavior is evidence of distress or an unmet need for help.

Assumption 3

When patients cannot meet their own needs they become distressed (Orlando, 1961). When patients become distressed they are dependent on the nurse for help. If patients are able to meet their own needs and follow prescribed activities unaided, they do not require the nurse's help. Therefore, nurses must be able to validate whether or not patients require their help at a given time (Orlando, 1961).

Assumption 4

The patient's behavior is meaningful. Although the behavior has a specific meaning to the patient this meaning is not self-evident. On the surface a patient's problem may look simple and the nurse may think she or he can apply some knowledge from another field to solve the problem. However, what becomes apparent from Orlando's (1961) theory is that the meaning of the patient's behavior is rarely what it appears; thus arbitrary solutions are seldom helpful. Consequently the nurse, after observing a patient's behavior, realizes that she or he does not understand the meaning without further exploration with the patient (Orlando, 1961).

Assumption 5

Patients are able and willing to communicate verbally (and nonverbally when unable to communicate verbally). Implicit in the theory is that it is most useful with patients who are able and willing to communicate verbally. Although it can be used with babies and comatose or unconscious patients it does rely heavily on verbal communications. If patients are unable to speak or are unconscious, nurses could enlist family or significant others to participate on the patient's behalf or rely on their own observations of nonverbal vocal behavior and/or nonverbal physiological manifestations in carrying out a deliberative nursing process (Schmieding, 1986).

Assumptions About Nurses

Assumption 1

The nurse's reaction to each patient is unique. According to Orlando (1961, 1972) each nurse's immediate reaction is based on how the nurse experiences her or his participation in the nurse-patient situation. The nurse never knows in advance what her or his reaction to the patient will be. Orlando notes that in each situation the nurse has to find out more about her or his own reaction and action in order to understand its particular meaning to the patient (Orlando, 1961).

Assumption 2

Nurses are responsible for helping patients avoid or alleviate distress. Because they are responsible to alleviate patients' distress or to help patients avoid distress nurses must focus on eliminating things that interfere with the patient's mental and physical comfort. Conversely, nurses should not add to the patient's distress (Orlando, 1961).

Assumption 3

The nurse's mind is the major tool for helping patients. Similar to Burr, Hill, Nye, and Reiss (1979), Orlando regards the nurse's mind as the chief vehicle for converting mental processes, perceived from an immediate situation, into action. What occurs in the mind is in large part a function of what occurs in the interaction. The nurse's mind, therefore, is the intervening variable between the nurse's unique perception and its conversion into action. Orlando (1961) notes that what a nurse automatically perceives or thinks is not as important as what the nurse does. What the nurse says or does is an outcome of the nurse's reaction in the situation. Thus, the nurse's behavior is influenced by the meaning the nurse attaches to the thought she or he has in the mind. Therefore, the nurse's mind, and its content, is the nurse's major tool. Orlando describes how the nurse should use her or his reaction in an exploratory way to find the meaning of the patient's behavior (Orlando, 1961). Orlando assumes that nurses are logical thinkers who can convert the content of their minds into actions that ultimately will benefit the patient.

Assumption 4

The nurse's use of automatic responses prevents the responsibility of nursing from being fulfilled. When a nurse acts without deliberations with the patient, the action often is not helpful because the nurse does not consider the patient's perception. Automatic personal responses are based on assumptions and are rarely reliable for decision making or action. Because the nurse's automatic response does not include the patient, communications between patient and nurse become unclear or stop (Orlando, 1961). The patient's distress or sense of helplessness continues because the nurse's action is based on reasons other than the patient's immediate need for help (Orlando, 1961).

Assumption 5

A nurse's practice is improved through self-reflection. The nurse's words and actions are the exclusive mode through which the patient is served. Therefore, the focus of improvement is on what nurses say and do and how these practices influence the process of care. As nurses comprehend how their practice helped or did not help the patient, this understanding comprises the material out of which nurses develop and improve their knowledge and skill in practice (Orlando, 1961). Self-reflection, as a method to improve a practitioner's practice, is supported by action science as developed by Argyris and Shön (1978).

Assumptions About
the Nurse-Patient Situation

Assumption 1

The nurse-patient situation is a dynamic whole. Because the patient and the nurse are people, they interact and a process occurs between them. In this process, what the nurse says and does affects the patient and what the patient says and does affects the nurse (Orlando, 1961). This process is unique for each situation. Orlando (1961) notes that when the nurse expresses her or his perceptions or thoughts as questions or wonderings it enables the patient to express the meaning the patient has of the nurse's expression. When nurses explore the meaning of the patient's behavior the patient is more willing to express her or his concerns. Once patients have been helped and trust the nurse, their communications are more spontaneous and explicit (Orlando, 1961).

Assumption 2

The phenomenon of the nurse-patient encounter represents a major source of nursing knowledge. The nurse's perception of a patient's behavior, and her or his subsequent thoughts and feelings, are objective and subjective data acquired through the nurse's direct experience with the patient. Although they require investigation, these data represent the knowledge base out of which the patient's plan of care will be developed.

Accepting these assumptions is prerequisite to the theory's acceptance. These assumptions are the foundation for the formulations of the interrelated concepts that constitute Orlando's theory.

3

Major Dimensions of the Theory

Theories allow a systematic way to look at the world in order to describe, explain, predict, and control it (Torres, 1990). Theories are invented to help people solve problems. In nursing, theories help the nurse make decisions and take actions in practice situations. A theory is an intellectual tool that directs one's focus of investigation or exploration of specific phenomena. It is like a map that picks out the most important parts of the phenomena (Barnum, 1990). Because it emphasizes certain aspects of a phenomenon it restricts the boundaries of inquiry (Dewey, 1938), thus ferreting out irrelevant data and making the processing of the remaining complex data more manageable. Therefore when nurses are caring for patients, theories help nurses select and organize direct patient observations and indirect patient data from records and reports to use in deciding their approach to a patient's care. Theories give nurses a sense of purpose and direction for their actions, and without their use patient outcomes are achieved on a hit-or-miss basis. When selecting a theory a nurse should assess its effectiveness in solving practice problems; the theory also should be easy to use.

Concepts are the building blocks of a theory; thus a theory contains a set of interrelated concepts. Concepts are mental images or ideas that come to mind when one observes the phenomenon of interest. They help one impose intellectual organization upon observations (Harré, 1989). They are ideas that one carries around in one's mind. For a theory to be useful to nursing practice it should contain a sufficient number of concepts for the nurse to use to comprehend complex phenomena. However, if a theory has too many concepts it is difficult to grasp the phenomenon. A theory's concepts are abstract; therefore they are inferred or indirectly observed. In nursing, the more abstract a concept, the more difficult it is to grasp its meaning, and thus, the more difficult to infer it empirically through patient observations.

An elaboration of the five major concepts of Orlando's theory illuminates their logical relationship and describes the nursing practice that results from the systematic use of the theory's concepts. Although the concepts are interrelated they are discussed separately here. Other secondary nursing concepts related to the theory's major concepts are integrated throughout the discussion.

Professional Nursing Function

Orlando (1961) believes that inadequate patient care was caused by the profession's lack of a clearly articulated nursing function. According to Orlando professional authority is derived from the profession's distinct function; therefore without this distinctiveness nursing practice cannot be autonomous because it lacks authority. Orlando (1961) thinks the lack of a distinct function has interfered with the development of a framework to evaluate the influence of the nurse's actions on patient outcomes.

Orlando formulated her concept of the nursing function by analyzing the outcomes of nurse-patient contacts in problematic situations. The context within which this concept evolved relates to Orlando's view of nursing, which focuses on the patient's immediate needs for help in the immediate experience. She states:

> Nursing . . . is responsive to individuals who suffer or anticipate a sense of helplessness; it is focused on the process of care in an immediate experience; it is concerned with providing direct assistance to individuals in whatever setting they are found for the purpose of avoiding, relieving, diminishing or curing the individual's sense of helplessness. (Orlando, 1972, p. 12)

According to Orlando (1961), helplessness, need, or stress originate from the patient's physical limitations, adverse reactions to the setting, and experiences that prevent the patient from communicating her or his needs. When a patient is ill or in some state of difficulty she or he often is unable to meet her or his own needs. *"Need is situationally defined as a requirement of the patient which, if supplied, relieves or diminishes his immediate distress or improves his immediate sense of adequacy or well-being"* (Orlando, 1961, p. 5). Therefore "learning how to understand what is happening between herself and the patient is the central core of the nurse's practice and comprises the basic framework for the help she gives to patients" (Orlando, 1961, p. 4).

The function of professional nursing is the principal organizing concept of Orlando's theory, which means it is the fundamental concept around which the theory's other concepts revolve. She envisions the nursing function as "finding out and meeting the patient's immediate needs for help" (Orlando, 1972, p. 20). The patient's "immediate needs for help" should not be confused with basic human needs. Basic needs are shared by all people, whereas the need for help is highly individualized and varied (Orlando, 1987). Orlando's conception of need is specific to *the help* a person requires in an immediate situation. The distinct function clarifies the nurse's role and guides inquiry by directing the nurse's focus to the patient's immediate experience. Thus, the patient's experience is the focal point of the nurse's investigation. According to Orlando (1972), the "distinct professional function is constant regardless of the patient's age, diagnosis or treatment, whether housed at home or in an institution or agency" (p. 20).

Orlando (1972) notes that at the onset of nurse-patient contact it is not known to the nurse whether the patient is in need of help. However, information is available through exploration with the patient for achieving a correct understanding of the patient's behavior and determining whether the patient is in need of help. If the patient is in need and the need for help is met by the nurse, the professional function has been fulfilled. Orlando (1972) describes the results in the following way: "The product of meeting the patient's immediate need for help is . . . 'improvement' in the immediate verbal and nonverbal behavior of the patient. This observable change allows the nurse to believe or disbelieve that her activity relieved, prevented or diminished the patient's sense of helplessness" (p. 21). In Orlando's theory both the aim and the end result of nursing are improvement in the patient's behavior.

Repetitious use of the concept—finding out and meeting the patient's immediate need for help—guides the nurse's investigation and makes the nurse sensitive to specific stimuli in nurse-patient situations. Finding out and meeting the patient's immediate needs for help becomes an acquired way of thinking; thus in each situation the nurse's underlying thought is, "Does the patient have an immediate need for help or not?" The nurse then explores her or his observations with the patient to confirm or refute an immediate need for help (Schmieding, 1987). Because it directs the nurse's focus to the patient this concept provides specific boundaries to the nurse's practice, thereby increasing intellectual efficiency and decreasing confusion. The nurse also can use the concept of function to decide whether an activity or task is non-nursing. The question to be answered is, "Does the activity help the nurse find out and meet the patient's immediate need for help?"

The concept of the nursing function, as articulated by Orlando, clearly establishes the nurse's accountability to the patient and provides an evaluative framework. Orlando (1972) stresses that evaluation must take place each time a nurse acts. Orlando (1972) considers that it is the nurse's direct responsibility to meet the patient's immediate need, either personally or by calling in the services of others. With the emphasis that Orlando places on the patient's immediate experience, it is logical that the patient's behavior is another major concept of her theory.

The Patient's Presenting Behavior

Orlando's theory focuses exclusively on understanding the complexities of problematic situations. Nursing practice is made up of frequent nurse-patient contacts in which patients may make remarks such as: "Can I have something for pain?" "I can't get out of bed!" "My baby is not getting enough to eat." "How long have you been a nurse?" or "Please pull down my blind." In these contacts it is not clear whether or not patients are experiencing distress or are in need of help. The nurse is responsible, and should be professionally prepared, to help patients communicate their need for help and to see that their immediate need is met. Because this identification of need is the foundation of the nurse-patient relationship, nurses must develop skills in exploring with patients the meaning of their verbal and nonverbal behavior (Orlando, 1961).

The discovery and meeting of patients' immediate needs for help are not straightforward. Patients often are unable to express the nature of their distress without the nurse's help. Orlando (1961) believes the reasons patients may not clearly communicate distress could be related to not knowing in a real sense how the nurse might help, as well as experiencing ambivalence about their dependency needs. Whatever the cause, the nurse must assume that the patient's behavior may indicate an unmet need for help unless the nurse has contrary evidence (Orlando, 1961). Therefore the nurse should view patients' behavior as not immediately understandable, but as a means to understanding. From her observations of practice Orlando (1961) formulated the following concept to guide the nurse's observation: *"The presenting behavior of the patient, regardless of the form in which it appears, may represent a plea for help"* (p. 40).

Patients' behavior can be manifested in the following forms: (a) verbal, such as asking a question, making a demand or request, or making a statement to the nurse; (b) nonverbal vocal, such as coughing, moaning, crying, and wheezing; and (c) nonverbal, such as tears in the eyes, skin color, pacing, reddened face, clenched fist, or physiological manifestations such as blood pressure and pulse (Orlando, 1961). Whatever the behavior, it causes the nurse to take notice. However, the initial behavior is unreliable for interpreting the meaning of patients' behavior because the behavior may *not* indicate that patients are distressed or the true nature of the distress. In other words, the behavior may not mean what it appears to mean. Therefore the nurse must be able to find out the meaning of the behavior and then determine the patient's immediate need for help.

Because the patient's behavior may be a cue or signal to the nurse, the patient's presenting behavior always should be explored. Orlando specifies that both the patient and the nurse participate in this exploratory communication process to identify the problem as well as the solution. She writes:

First, *the nurse must take the initiative in helping the patient express the specific meaning of his behavior in order to ascertain his distress.* Second, *she must help the patient explore the distress in order to ascertain the help he requires for his [immediate] need [for help] to be met.* (Orlando, 1961, p. 26)

Because the patient's behavior stimulates the nurse's perceptions it becomes the starting point of the nurse's investigation. According to Orlando, the nurse's perception of the patient's presenting behavior forms the basis of the nurse's thoughts and feelings. This perception is discussed in the next section.

Immediate Reaction

The nurse's direct observation of the patient's presenting behavior is the basis of the nurse's perceptions, thoughts, and feelings, which occur in an automatic, almost instantaneous sequence (Orlando, 1972). This observation represents the first data and the only resource the nurse can use in understanding the meaning of the patient's behavior. The nurse's reaction, stimulated by the patient's behavior, comes from the nurse's past experiences and knowledge, which combine with the nurse's understanding of the immediate situation to produce the nurse's unique reaction.

According to Orlando (1961) a nursing situation is comprised of the patient's behavior, the nurse's reaction, and the nurse's action. The interaction of these is called the nursing process. To describe the process more specifically Orlando (1972) identified four distinct items in any person's action process and described the sequence of their occurrence. She notes:

These separate items reside within an individual and at any given moment occur in the following automatic, sometimes instantaneous, sequence: (1) The person perceives with any one of his five sense organs an object or objects; (2) The perceptions stimulate automatic thought; (3) Each thought stimulates an automatic feeling; and (4) Then the person acts. (Orlando, 1972, p. 25)

The first three items are defined as the person's immediate reaction and cannot be observed; only the action, which is what the person says and conveys nonverbally, can be observed.

Orlando (1961) views the immediate reaction as unique to each situation and notes that in a nursing situation what a nurse perceives, thinks, and feels about the patient's behavior reflects the nurse's individuality. She explains that the nurse's automatic thoughts about the perception reflect the nurse's meaning or interpretation attached to the perception. From the patient's viewpoint the nurse's meanings may or may not be correct. However, regardless of the extent of their accuracy, the perceptions that provoke the nurse's thoughts are communications from the patient and as such are "raw" data for the nurse to use in her or his investigation of the patient's behavior. Orlando (1961) notes that if the nurse was preoccupied with the application of principles this preoccupation would condition the nurse's first thoughts.

Orlando views the nurse's appropriate use of the immediate reaction as critical to understanding the meaning of the patient's behavior. Orlando formulated a deliberative nursing process to help the nurse use her or his immediate reactions.

Deliberative Nursing Process

Orlando's (1961) deliberative nursing process[1] formulations reflect her view of the nurse-patient situation as a dynamic whole; the patient's behavior affects the nurse and the nurse's behavior (action) affects the patient. In developing her theory Orlando carefully analyzed nurse-patient contacts to determine what nurse action resulted in a positive patient outcome as well as what contributed to negative outcomes. Nurse actions with positive results were called a deliberative nursing process, whereas nurse actions that produced negative patient outcomes were called automatic personal responses.

According to Orlando (1972) the use of a deliberative nursing action requires that a shared communication process occur between the nurse and the patient in order to determine: (a) the meaning of the patient's behavior, (b) the help required by the patient, and (c) whether the patient was helped by the nurse's action.

To comprehend this approach it is necessary to explain Orlando's (1972) conception of a person's action process. In a person-to-person contact each person experiences an immediate reaction that contains the person's perception about the observed behavior of another

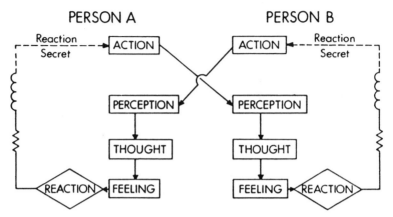

Figure 3.1. The action process in a person-to-person contact functioning in secret. The perceptions, thoughts, and feelings of each individual are not directly available to the perception of the other individual through the observable action.

SOURCE: Orlando, 1972, p. 26. Reprinted by permission.

person, the thought about the perception, and a feeling associated with the thought. These items remain a secret from the other person unless the first individual openly discloses them. Only the first individual's action is available to the other person (see Figures 3.1 and 3.2 to visualize these processes). In other words, if a nurse makes a statement to the patient and does not share what perception, thought, or feeling formed the basis of the action, the patient remains unaware of them. This sequential process, whether disclosed or not, continues throughout the entire contact.

Although the separation of perceptions, thoughts, and feelings is extremely difficult, this process helps nurses see how one aspect of their reaction affects the other aspects (Orlando, 1961). Orlando developed guidelines (1972) that specify how a person should use the content of her or his immediate reaction in a deliberative way, through open disclosure, to achieve a helpful patient outcome. The guidelines include the following: (a) in a situation a person verbally states to the other person any or all the items in her or his immediate reaction, (b) the stated item must be expressed as self-designated, and (c) the person asks the other person to verify or correct the item verbally expressed. In a nurse-patient contact Orlando's delibera-

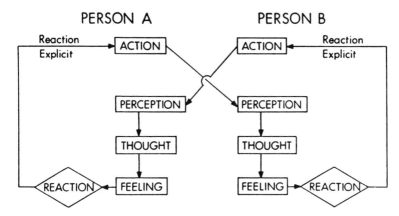

Figure 3.2. The action process in a person-to-person contact functioning by open disclosure. The perceptions, thoughts, and feelings of each individual are directly available to the perception of the other individual through the observable action.

SOURCE: Orlando, 1972, p. 26. Reprinted by permission.

tive nursing process can be described as follows: Whatever the nurse perceives about the patient with any one of the five sense organs and thinks and feels about this perception must, at least in part, be verbally expressed as self-designated to the patient and then asked about. Only the person involved in the person-to-person contact can verify ownership of the items. An example would be, "I noticed your face got red as you talked about your doctor (a visual perception stated as self-designated). I thought you might be angry with him (thought about the perception stated as self-designated). Could that be or not (requests verification or correction)?" The nurse continues this process until she or he observes and verifies, with the patient, improvement in the patient's verbal and nonverbal behavior.

The nurse who uses this type of action is more likely to find out and meet the patient's immediate needs for help because when the nurse expresses her or his immediate reaction the patient also is more likely to do so (Orlando, 1972). The nurse's expression of his or her reaction minimizes the opportunity for the nurse to make assumptions and increases the chance to correct or verify the nurse's private interpretations of the patient's action. Both people have a better understanding of how the other experienced the immediate situation (Orlando, 1972). "Failure to impose the entire discipline on the nurse's own process at least some of the time with any one person may result in misinterpretation of actions on both sides" (Pelletier, 1968, p. 4).

Orlando (1961) provided helpful guidlines for the nurse to use in expressing her or his immediate reactions in a deliberate, exploratory way. To explore the observed behavior, she wrote, "*any observation [perception] shared and explored with the patient is immediately useful in ascertaining and meeting his need or finding out that he is not in need at that time*" (Orlando, 1961, pp. 35-36). An example is, "I notice tears in your eyes. Could that be or not?" Because the patient is more likely to agree with the correctness of the nurse's perception, its use is more efficient than first exploring thoughts (Orlando, 1961). Efficiency is important because the longer patients are frustrated in getting help, the more distressful their presenting behavior and the more obscure its meaning (Orlando, 1961).

The nurse's automatic thoughts about perceptions also can be used to explore the patient's behavior. Because the nurse's thoughts about her or his perception are likely to be inadequate, incorrect, or only partially correct, the nurse should explore their validity. In describing the nurse's use of the immediate thoughts, Orlando (1961) wrote, "*The nurse does not assume that any aspect of her reaction* [here meaning thought] *to the patient is correct, helpful or appropriate until she checks the validity of it in exploration with the patient*" (p. 56). Therefore the nurse should use her or his thoughts deliberatively, namely through exploration for their relevance to the present situation. In understanding the nature of thoughts Orlando (1961) cautions that a nurse is more likely to assume that her or his thoughts about a perception are correct if they are not tentatively formulated as questions or wonderings. When the nurse states her or his thoughts as a tentative possibility the patient is more likely to respond with her or his own negative reaction. For example: "I saw you close your eyes when I started to change your colostomy bag. I thought you might be frightened about having to learn how to do this yourself. Could that be or not?"

After the thought about the perception the nurse experiences a feeling, which may be positive or negative. Regardless of whether the feeling is negative or positive it can be as useful as perceptions and thoughts, provided the patient has an opportunity to respond to it (Orlando, 1961). When the nurse explores her or his feeling

Orlando (1972) proposes that the nurse also state the perception that provoked the thought rather than stating only the feeling. For example, if the nurse was angry because the patient kept asking for a bedpan and the nurse thought the patient did not need it, the nurse would state: "I get angry when you keep asking for the bedpan because I don't think you need it. Am I right or not?" If the nurse does not resolve her or his feelings with the patient these same feelings may occur again when in contact with the patient. In addition, if these feelings are not expressed and explored they may show in the nurse's nonverbal behavior (Orlando, 1961).

Determining the meaning of the patient's behavior and identifying the patient's immediate need for help do not end the nurse's responsibility to the patient. Therefore in each situation the nurse initiates an exploratory process to ascertain how the patient is affected by what she or he says or does (Orlando, 1961). Orlando stresses that it is not the nurse's activity that is evaluated but rather its effects upon the patient. Only through this evaluative process can a nurse become aware of how and whether her or his action helped the patient.

Unlike the current usage of the term *nursing process,* Orlando's deliberative nursing process is *not* a linear process of assessing, diagnosing, planning, implementing, and evaluating, with each step following the other in unvaried sequence. Rather the deliberative nursing process is a "muddy," serial, back-and-forth process because it has elements of continuous reflection as the nurse attempts to understand the patient's meaning of the behavior and what help the patient needs from the nurse in order to be helped. These responses are stimulated by the nurse's unfolding awareness of the particulars of the individual situation (Orlando, 1961). Orlando thinks the use of the deliberative nursing process helps the nurse fulfill the nursing function because the nurse finds out and meets the patient's immediate needs for help. However, when a nurse uses an automatic personal response the patient's distress is not relieved because communication between them becomes unclear (Orlando, 1961).

Automatic Personal Responses

Orlando (1961) asserts that people's automatic reactions and actions, inherent in a nursing situation, are likely to cause unclear communication, which creates a situational conflict. Therefore understanding the nature of automatic responses is necessary to recognize the problems associated with their use. This understanding helps the nurse to avoid the pitfall of having a "ready" answer or solution to the problem at hand. Orlando (1961) characterizes automatic personal responses as being decided upon without the patient's perception of the situation and for reasons other than the patient's immediate need for help.

Orlando (1961) observed that automatic responses contribute to inadequate communications because items of a person's immediate reaction are withheld from the other person. Thus the first person makes assumptions about the situation that are never verified or corrected. For the nurse these assumptions form an unreliable basis for decision making and action because the patient does not participate in the process. Orlando (1972) specifies why automatic responses, which are contrary to the nurse's use of a deliberative process of action, are not helpful:

1. When a nurse withholds his or her immediate reaction, the patient cannot verify or correct it. This withholding allows the patient to make assumptions about the nurse's verbal and nonverbal behavior.
2. If the nurse's response is not stated as self-designated the patient is allowed to make assumptions about the origin of what is heard (the use of "we" does not clearly provide the origin).
3. If the nurse's response is not in the form of a question the other person may not feel free to correct or verify what was heard. As a result neither person in the contact knows the immediate reaction of the other; therefore each is left with an unverified understanding of the other's action (Orlando, 1972).

Figure 3.1 reinforces this description.

Orlando (1961) stresses that actions based on the nurse's conclusion, arrived at without deliberation with the patient, often are not helpful. Thus, an action carried out automatically, without the patient's participation, could be correct but ineffective in helping the patient (Orlando, 1961).

The nurse's experience of the immediate situation is not sufficient to understand a patient's presenting behavior. Rather, in each nurse-patient experience a deliberative process of inquiry is needed to prevent the use of automatic responses and activities.

Orlando's deliberative nursing process is an integral part of her formulations, thus making it a practical theory to use. The simplicity of this deliberative approach, however, disguises the complexity of its use. As with any skill the use of the deliberative nursing process must be developed through practice. Self-reflection through the analysis of one's action process helps the nurse recognize when she or he does not act in a deliberative manner.

Improvement

The last major concept in Orlando's theory is improvement in the patient's behavior. If the nurse's activity meets the patient's immediate needs for help, the patient's behavior improves from what it had been; if the patient's behavior does not change the nursing function has not been met.

> In both situations the results are available immediately after the activity is performed. . . . The product of meeting the patient's immediate need for help is . . . "improvement" in the verbal and nonverbal behavior of the patient. This observable change allows the nurse to believe or disbelieve that her activity relieved, prevented or diminished the patient's sense of helplessness. (Orlando, 1972, p. 21)

When the patient's behavior has improved the situation loses its problematic character; the equilibrium changes to a unified whole. The nurse uses this concept of improvement to evaluate whether her or his activity has produced a change in the patient's condition (the product of professional nursing). Namely, did the nurse help the patient communicate clearly and did this process help direct how the patient's need for help would be met? Orlando (1961) believes improvement is relative to what condition existed when the nurse and patient started the process, the length of their relationship, what they were able to accomplish, and whether the patient notes an increased sense of well-being. She asserts that the nurse's "own individuality and that of the patient require that she go through this each time she is called upon to render service to those who need her" (Orlando, 1961, p. 91).

Orlando (1961) states that she did not deal with long-range nursing goals. She believes the process of helping a patient occurs in the immediate situation and the outcome for the patient depends on the help provided in that immediate experience.

The nature of the concepts in this nursing process theory demonstrates that Orlando envisions nursing as a creative process that begins and ends in the patient's immediate experience. Her formulations of a person's action process and her prescriptions on how to use the elements of the nurse's immediate reaction make it a practical nursing practice theory.

Note

1. *Deliberative nursing process* was renamed *nursing process discipline* in 1972. *Deliberative nursing process* is used in this book to provide consistency.

4

The Theory's Propositions and Implied Research

"Propositions are statements of relationships between concepts in the theoretical system" (Kim, 1983, p. 11). "Until one has propositional statements about the relationship between the concepts one does not have a usable theory" (Burr et al., 1979, p. 52). Propositions state the theory's concepts in an associational or causal way that indicates that the relationship can be measured. Thus propositions provide a means for developing hypotheses so the theory can be tested through research. Without research, the theory's influence on nursing practice can only be assumed. It is only through research that these assumptions can be confirmed or refuted. It is through research that a theory can be further developed or refined.

Orlando did not formulate explicit propositions of her theory; however, propositional statements can be derived from her concepts. Following each proposition, research implied by the proposition is suggested.

Proposition 1: There is a relationship between the *patient's presenting behavior* and the presence of patient distress *(an immediate need for help)*.

When patients have an unmet need for help they become distressed (Orlando, 1961). This distress is manifested through their behavior. Behaviors can be conveyed to the nurse through verbal and nonverbal communications.

A research study could be undertaken to categorize the following types of verbal communication to the nurse: questions, complaints, and requests. Nurses trained in the use of Orlando's deliberative nursing process would explore the meaning to the patient of the verbal communications and categorize results into types of distress or no distress. Although the patient's distress is unique, knowledge about the type of behavior that is most often used by patients to communicate certain types of distress, and their associated need for help, would be a helpful resource to nurses for exploration of similar situations in the future. Also, these findings would be useful for developing further research, and for educational purposes.

Proposition 2: There is a relationship between a nurse's use of Orlando's *distinct nursing function* and the nurse's ability to recognize the need for inquiry *(deliberative nursing process)* into the meaning of the *patient's presenting behavior.*

Dewey (1938) and Kuhn (1970) both believe that the use of an organizing principle (such as Orlando's function of nursing) allows a person to recognize a situation as problematic. Early recognition of a patient's immediate need for help is important because the longer the patient experiences distress, the greater the distress becomes and the more obscure the patient's behavior (Orlando, 1961). The more obscure the behavior, the more difficult it is for the nurse to find out what the patient is distressed about. According to Orlando (1961) the treatment and prevention of a disease proceeds best when patients are not distressed.

Research could be designed to examine differences in nurse responses in patient encounters between nurses who use "finding out and meeting the patient's immediate need for help" and nurses who use a different theory and/or no nursing theory. Implied in this research is the relationship between the nurse's immediate reaction to a patient's verbal request and the use of all or part of the immediate reaction in the nurse's response.

Proposition 3: The more competent the nurse is in labeling her or his perceptions, thoughts, and feelings *(immediate reaction)*, the more apt she or he is to find out *(deliberative nursing process)* the nature of the patient's distress.

According to Orlando (1961), although it is difficult to separate the items of the immediate reaction, it is important to do so because it helps the nurse understand how the items influence each other. If the nurse does not understand the basis of her or his process of action it is difficult for the nurse to use the immediate reaction effectively in exploration of the patient's behavior. Orlando (1961) believes the exploration of any part of the nurse's reaction is immediately helpful in determining the patient's need for help.

A research study that includes the education of nurses in the use of Orlando's theory could be designed to compare nurses' identification of patient distress and associated need for help between nurses who can accurately separate their immediate reaction with nurses unable to do so. A secondary research component in this study could be to identify types of patient behavior that are more likely associated with the nurse's ability or inability to accurately separate the items of her or his immediate reaction.

Proposition 4: If the nurse explores her or his *immediate reaction* with the patient the patient's distress is lessened *(improvement)*.

The major aim of Orlando's (1961) theory is to bring about improvement in the patient's verbal and nonverbal behavior, thus improving the nursing care of patients. If the patient's immediate needs for help are not found out and met, the patient's condition remains the same or worsens. A patient's condition might be seriously threatened if the distress is not relieved. After the nurse's action, the nurse is able to determine immediately whether the distress was relieved by observing changes in the patient's verbal and nonverbal behavior. Research that compares patient outcomes when nurses explore and when they do not explore the patient's presenting behavior could be used to test the theory.

In addition to research on the effects of improvement in the patient's immediate behavior, other indicators reflecting improvement might be studied. For example, experimental research could compare randomly assigned patients who have deliberative nursing care with those who have automatic nursing care by measuring patient levels of anxiety, depression, or helplessness after each shift. This study would measure the immediate influence of nursing on patients. A variety of standardized instruments are available to measure these concepts. Patient distress also could be operationalized as increased dependence, which could be measured with standardized instruments.

> Proposition 5: The nurse's use of the *deliberative nursing process* will be less costly than the nurse's use of *automatic personal responses* (a secondary concept of the theory).

Because automatic actions are based on conclusions arrived at independently of the patient they most often are not helpful, as they do not consider the patient's perception of the situation. Because the nurse arbitrarily applies a solution to what she or he thinks the patient's problem is, that solution often is ineffective and therefore costly in terms of the nurse's time, materials, and drugs. It also may prolong the patient's hospitalization or use of ambulatory services. Recently, reducing health-care costs has been a major national goal. Therefore the nurse's use of a deliberative nursing process might be both effective and efficient.

One research question would be, "Are nurses who use a deliberative nursing process approach to explore the patient's behavior more likely to reduce costs than those who use automatic personal actions?" The study could measure such costs as length of stay or health-care visits, use of analgesics and hypnotics, and nursing contact hours.

> Proposition 6: Patients experiencing repeated *improvement* as the result of *deliberative nursing* will have positive cumulative effects.

Orlando (1961) often refers to the cumulative effects of repeated patient improvement as the result of deliberative nursing. She notes that although improvement is always relative to the patient's condition at the start of the nurse-patient contact, these repeated improvements may positively contribute to the patient's improved self-care. At another time she notes that improvement is related to the length of the nurse-patient contact and to what they accomplish in each contact. Even though the changes might be small they may have cumulative value (Orlando, 1961).

Research could be designed to measure the degree of self-care competence in colostomy care on discharge in two groups of patients, one receiving deliberative nursing and the other nondeliberative nursing care. A research question for obstetrical nursing is, "Do primiparous women feel more confident about self- and newborn care at discharge when they have received deliberative nursing care versus nondeliberative nursing care?" Also, a researcher could compare patients' sense of self-care confidence immediately prior to discharge in cohorts of patients receiving deliberative and nondeliberative care.

Orlando's propositions provide a way to study systematically the elements of her theory. These proposed research studies would provide information to further assess the theory's internal validity as well as to determine how the nurse's use of the theory influences the outcome of the patient's condition.

5

Research of the Theory

Whereas the understanding of a professional discipline is gained through its theories, to a great extent, knowledge of that discipline is gained through research (Walker, 1992). One way to expand nursing knowledge is through research of its theories. According to Barnum (1990), for a nursing theory to be relevant it must meet three criteria: (a) it addresses essential nursing issues, (b) it contributes to knowledge development in nursing, and (c) it has research potential. Research tests a theory's description or explanation as well as providing a body of related knowledge (Barnum, 1990).

In nursing, research of a theory serves to develop and refine theory and to improve practice. As new knowledge is implemented into practice it stimulates further research. The theory-research-practice process continues in a circular fashion and results in improvement and/or refinement of practice.

Because nursing is a practice discipline it has an obligation to society to generate new knowledge continually so nursing care can be based on validated research. Tradition, habit, or intuition are insufficient as the basis of practice (Torres, 1990). The use of theories in practice, and the research of them, provides the means for a profession to progress; it also helps fulfill the profession's obligation to society.

Research of Orlando's theory began at Yale University shortly after the theory's development. These studies are hallmarks in clinical nursing research. Some investigators used elements of Orlando's theory without acknowledgment; some of these are included in the bibliography. In this chapter clinical research is briefly summarized, according to major focus areas, followed by a section on the theory's use in education and administration.

Studies on Patient's Presenting Behavior

In a study to determine whether patients clearly and adequately expressed their need for help, Elder (1963) found that initially patients did not adequately communicate their need and that the patient's behavior was unreliable for assessing the patient's degree of discomfort. Research on postpartum patients' perceptions of needs by Faulkner (1963) revealed that the patient's expression of one need for help may have several associated needs. She also found that patients rarely summon nurses for emotional needs. Gowan and Morris (1964) found that 81% of postoperative patients had other needs that were unexpressed because "the nurse was perceived as too busy," "hated to bother nurse," or thought the "nurse would disapprove."

Fischelis (1963) conducted a study to determine whether nurses who labeled patients explored the patient's behavior and whether the labels led to beneficial activities. She found that nurses who labeled patients had not explored the meaning of the patient's behavior. Interviews with patients revealed that none of the nurses' explanations of the patient's behavior were correct and that the nurses' activities had not benefited the patient.

Studies on the Effectiveness of Deliberative Nursing

Four studies were designed to examine whether deliberative nursing relieved specific patient distress. In an experimental study of patients experiencing sleeplessness, Gillis (1976) found that patients in the experimental group used fewer sleep medications than those in the control group. Three studies have indicated that deliberative nursing reduced distress from pain (Barron, 1966; Bochnak, Rhymes,

& Leonard, 1962, also reported in Bochnak, 1963; Tarasuk [Bochnak], Rhymes, & Leonard, 1965). The major findings of these studies were that patients receiving deliberative nursing used fewer pain medications, and experienced greater speed and degree of pain relief than did those patients receiving other forms of nursing.

Cameron (1962, 1963) found that nurses using questions to clarify and interpret were more effective in removing barriers that interfered with patient comfort or capability than questions seeking factual information. In a study of patient-initiated interactions, Dye (1963a, 1963b) found that patient distress was more often relieved by deliberative nursing. The results also indicated that most nursing actions were nondeliberative and that adverse reactions to the setting were the major cause of patient distress.

Studies documenting the positive effects of deliberative nursing actions on specific patient physiological outcomes are found in the upcoming studies.

In two pilot studies of patients admitted to an emergency room and to a psychiatric hospital, Anderson, Mertz, and Leonard (1965; also reported in Mertz, 1963) found a statistically significant difference in patient vital signs between patients receiving deliberative and nondeliberative nursing.

In an exploratory study of patients scheduled for gynecological elective surgery, Elms's (1964) results revealed that pulse rate showed a significant decrease as the result of deliberative nursing and more of these patients indicated that their distress was relieved by the nurse's approach. In a larger study using the same design and type of patient a difference did not exist in pulse rate but more patients in the experimental group cited nursing as a factor in distress relief than did those in the control group (Elms & Leonard, 1966).

The use of a deliberative nursing process with gynecological patients was studied by Dumas and her colleagues. In three experimental studies, one of which was a pilot, Dumas and Leonard (1963; also reported in Dumas, 1963) found the incidence of postoperative vomiting to be significantly less in patients whose nurse used deliberative nursing. Patients whose distress was not relieved preoperatively tended to vomit more postoperatively. However, contradictory results were found in a subsequent study on the same unit, but with a different nurse providing care (Dumas, Anderson, & Leonard, 1965). In another experimental study Dumas and Johnson [Anderson] (1972) measured the effects of a deliberative nursing process on seven variables associated with postoperative recovery. The stress level of patients who received deliberative nursing preoperatively was significantly lower than that of patients who did not. However, little difference was found between the two groups on the other indicators of recovery. Type of surgery was thought to be a significant confounding variable. Studying the incidence of vomiting in general postoperative patients, Rhymes (1964) found that the difference between patients who did not vomit or need catherization was related to deliberative nursing care.

In a study of patients in labor Tryon (1962; also reported in Tryon & Leonard, 1964) found that patients who participated in the preoperative plans had more effective enema results than those who did not participate. This finding lends some support to Orlando's theory that automatic activities, even though prescribed, often are not effective if the patient's reaction to the activity has not been considered. In a second study Tryon (1966) postulated that a deliberative nursing approach to routine "support" measures would increase patient participation; the results were inconclusive.

The next two studies tested the influence of deliberative nursing on physiological measurements other than vital signs. Using electively hospitalized medical patients Pride (1968) tested the causal connection between experimental nursing, friendly unfocused nursing, and "no approach" on patient stress, as measured by urine potassium and the IPAT anxiety scale, a physiochemical index of patient welfare. Pride found that urine potassium was lower in patients receiving experimental nursing than for patients receiving other forms of nursing. However, there was no relationship between patient's level of anxiety and type of nursing. Clausen [Cameron] (1983) found breast-feeding mothers who received deliberative nursing care exhibited higher level functioning of the milk ejection reflex than those who did not.

Research related to the care of children was the focus of the next two studies. Wolfer and Visintainer (1975) found that children who received deliberative nursing care prior to minor surgery had less upset behavior, were more cooperative, and had fewer postsurgery adjustment problems than children who did not. When comparing parents' knowledge of illness, care prescribed, and compliance with treatment, Thibaudeau and Reidy (1977) found that mothers who had received deliberative nursing, as compared with those who had not, had significantly more knowledge of illness and complications and complied more fully with the prescribed treatment.

Characteristics of Nurses
Who Use Deliberative Nursing

With adult cancer patients Ponte (1988) correlated primary nurses'
use of empathy skill and their use of Orlando's deliberative process.
A positive relationship was found between empathy skills and nurses'
use of a deliberative nursing process. Surprisingly, these primary
nurses scored low both on use of empathy skills and deliberative
nursing process.

Education and Administration Research

In addition to the previously mentioned research by Orlando
(1972), investigators have used Orlando's theory in nursing education and administration. Haggerty (1987) applied Orlando's theory
to the analysis of student nurses' responses to videotapes of patients
with differing distress behaviors and found that deliberative responses were not associated with type of educational program, but
were related to the type of patient distress.

Schmieding (1988) adapted Orlando's theory to the study of nurse
administrators' actions and found that in the majority administrators did not view situations posed to them by their staff as problematic, their feelings in the situation were overwhelmingly negative,
and they would act without further investigation. Subsequent research by Schmieding revealed that (a) nurses preferred that their
supervisor use exploratory actions with them, but the majority thought
their supervisor would use non-exploratory actions (1990b); (b) head
nurses seldom involved staff nurses in the problem-solving process
(1990a); and (c) a relationship was found between the head nurse's
response to a staff nurse and the staff nurse's response to patients
(1992).

Conclusion

These research findings lend some support to the validity of
Orlando's theory but further research, with stronger controls on
threats to internal validity and larger, randomly assigned samples,
should be developed. The use of Orlando's theory could provide a
means for increasing the influence of nursing on positive patient
outcomes.

6

Application to Practice

"One of the most important tests of a theory is its applicability in practice" (Barnum, 1990, p. 19). Orlando's theory is characterized as a practice theory that provides a framework to guide nurses' actions. A theory's language can influence its use. If the language is too abstract or esoteric nurses will have difficulty clearly understanding it and applying it to their practice. Orlando uses language nurses can readily understand and use in everyday practice.

According to Barnum, "the function of theory is to guide practice and to direct the mind-set of nurses. If it fails to do that, it is useless" (Barnum, 1990, p. 69). The ultimate criterion of a practice theory is whether the patient is helped through its use. Some criteria for selecting a practice theory are: (a) Does it provide conceptual direction to the nurse about how to use it to help the patient? (b) Can the nurse verify through empirical observations of the patient that the theory's use influenced the outcome? (c) Can it be incorporated into the nurse's mind-set and become an integral part of the nurse's practice?

Orlando's theory focuses the nurse's mind-set to the patient's immediate experience and emphasizes that only the patient can verify what he or she is experiencing. Orlando's theory is a process rather than a content theory, which becomes integrated into the nurse's total practice. Thus, a nurse does not have to stop and think, "Should I apply Orlando's theory in this case?" Rather it is a theory nurses consistently use with all patients and its concept of improvement enables nurses to verify their results immediately by observing changes in the patient's behavior.

The four cases in this section are four brief examples of situations where nurses used Orlando's deliberative process. The first three have been previously published (Schmieding, 1986). The last case is presented in a nursing process record form, designed by Orlando (1972), which depicts the nurse's action process. The examples are representative of situations where nurses feel frustrated, label patients, react against patients, or feel a concern for patients.

A 78-year-old man with compromised circulation caused by Raynaud's disease had recent skin grafts to his foot that were not healing as rapidly as expected. When his primary nurse was about to change his foot dressing she noticed that the patient had eaten only bites of his lunch (presenting behavior). The nurse's first two nursing actions were automatic personal responses that failed to help the patient express his distress. She said, "Didn't you like the food?" The patient replied, "It was OK." The nurse responded, "Then why didn't you eat it?" The patient responded, "I didn't feel hungry." The nurse was feeling frustrated and stopped to clarify what she was thinking and feeling. She then said, "I feel frustrated. The reason I asked why you didn't eat more was that I'm concerned that your skin graft won't properly heal if you do not eat enough protein. Can you understand my frustration?" The gentleman abruptly looked up at the nurse and said, "Gee, I didn't think anyone around here cared for an old man like me [the patient's distress]. Bring back the food and I'll try to eat more." Within a short time the patient had eaten all the food on the tray and, thereafter, continued to eat the food brought to him. His wound began to steadily heal and he was discharged within 1 week.

Referring to patients by behavioral terms or diagnostic labels can adversely influence the patient's care because the nurse bases her or his action on assumptions about the patient's label rather than on the patient's immediate behavior. The following case conveys how basing action on patient labels might interfere with individualized care.

A 62-year-old woman, diagnosed as schizophrenic, was admitted to a gynecology unit for uterine bleeding. The head nurse expressed concerns to her supervisor about caring for "schizophrenics" because nurses on the unit didn't know how to talk to this type of patient. The supervisor assured the head nurse that, as with other patients, the nurse's exploration of her or his immediate reaction with the patient was most effective in determining what help this patient needed. Shortly after the conversation the head nurse heard the patient yelling, "Don't take my blood, don't take my blood!" (presenting behavior). When the head nurse entered the room three people were assuring the patient that they were not trying to hurt her, but that they needed to test her blood to find out what was causing her illness (automatic actions based on their assumption that the patient thought they wanted to hurt her). The head nurse stepped to the patient's side and said, "I'd like to know why you are saying, 'Don't take my blood' " (exploring the head nurses's perception). The patient looked up, hesitated a moment, and then, pointing at the lab technician, resident, and staff nurse, said, "You, you, and you, get out." Then, pointing to the head nurse, she said, "You sit down and stay." The patient revealed to the head nurse that she was afraid the test would require too much blood and only make her weaker than she already was (the distress). After being assured that the test required only a little blood the patient consented to have the blood drawn.

Another incident occurred with the above patient when low census on two units required that the patients on both units be placed in one. Nurses on one unit told the head nurse it would be too upsetting to move the schizophrenic patient, and therefore, the patients from the other unit should be transferred to accommodate this patient even though there were more patients on the other unit. The head nurse agreed with this plan only if the nurse first validated this assumption with the patient. The nurse explained the problem to the patient and explored the assumption by stating, "The nurses and I think it would be too upsetting to you to move. Would it be?" The patient replied, "That's the problem! Get the wheelchair, honey, I'm ready to move." These two situations convey that Orlando's theory is useful in clinical nursing as well as for making administrative decisions.

Nurses are human, and thus at times have negative personal reactions toward patients that interfere with their ability to help those patients. Often these reactions are based on assumptions about the patient's behavior on which the nurse has placed a value judgment. If these thoughts are withheld, the patient is left to make her or his interpretation about the nurse's verbal and nonverbal behavior. In the following situation several nurses had negative reactions to the patient; one nurse expressed and explored her feeling to the patient and found out that her interpretation of the patient's behavior was incorrect.

A 39-year-old diabetic patient who was 4 months pregnant was admitted with vomiting. She spoke only when spoken to and remained in bed even though she could be up (presenting behavior). She said she had vomited, but the nurses had not observed it. During reports nurses speculated, "I don't think she really is vomiting" and "I don't think she really wants this baby." These remarks were passed from shift to shift and eventually these speculations were passed on as facts even though no one had confirmed them with the patient. One nurse was shocked to learn that the patient did not want her baby. Although apprehensive, the nurse decided to express her feeling to the patient. She stated, "I'm shocked because I hear you don't want this baby. Is that true?" Immediately the patient's eyes began to well over with tears and she sobbed, "That's not true. I want the baby, it's just that I'm afraid I'll die in labor [the patient's distress]. Fifteen years ago when my other child was born I wasn't diabetic." The nurse was stunned by the patient's remark and asked, "Does your doctor or anyone know of this?" The patient replied, "No, I thought if I told people they would think I was a hysterical woman." The patient then agreed to discuss this with both her doctor and her family. Nurses on the unit, when hearing about this, became sympathetic toward the patient. It must be emphasized that the misunderstanding might not have happened if the first nurse who had a negative reaction would have explored her or his assumption with the patient.

The last situation involves a 67-year-old man with terminal carcinoma of the lung. His condition was steadily deteriorating as evidenced by increased cyanosis and dyspnea. Radiation treatment was being done only for palliative purposes. While the patient was being transferred to the stretcher for treatment his dyspnea and cyanosis increased, whereupon he was returned to bed and his oxygen was increased. The nurse was concerned about how she could help this patient. The nurse's action processes are recorded in the nursing process record shown in Table 6.1. It dramatically shows how a nurse can help relieve distress in a dying patient.

TABLE 6.1 Nursing Process Record

Perception of or About the Patient	Thought and/or Feeling About the Perception	Said and/or Did to, With, or for the Patient
Patient staring into space. One arm over forehead. Tightly holding my hand.	I thought he was frightened. I felt concern for him.	"I think you're feeling frightened; is that so?"
"Yes." Then he sighed. Tightly holding my hand.	I thought it might help him to talk about his fears.	"I think it would be helpful if you talked about your fears. Could you?"
"I'm thinking about being sick." Removes arm from forehead.	I don't think I know what this means to him.	"Could you tell me more about what that means to you?"
"I'm scared because I know I'm not going to get better." Continues to hold my hand, but less tightly.	I thought he was right and that I needed to let him talk more about it. I felt sad.	"I think you're right. Can you talk more about it?"
"Well, I've asked God to speed it up."	My thought was that he made God part of his life.	"It sounds like God is part of your life. Do you feel that way?"
"Yes, he is always there." Less dyspnic and less cyanotic. Releases hand and folds both arms over chest.	I wonder if he wants to talk more about this or if he wants to rest.	"I'm wondering if there is anything else you'd like to say."
"No, I'd just like to rest for a while." He closed his eyes and was asleep in 5 minutes.		

SOURCE: Orlando, 1972.

Conclusion

Orlando's theory remains one of the most effective practice theories. It is appealing because it clearly describes what nurses perceive as "good nursing." Nurses participated in the theory's development by allowing their practice to be observed. They validated Orlando's categorization of nursing situations into "good" and "bad" nursing. Nurses know what good nursing is, and Orlando's theory provides the means to help nurses achieve this excellence in practice.

Glossary

Automatic activities
Automatic activities are those decided upon by the nurse for reasons other than the patient's immediate need (Orlando, 1961).

Automatic personal response
An automatic personal response is defined as the withholding of the items of a person's immediate reaction from the other person (Orlando, 1972).

*Deliberative nursing process (renamed "*nursing process discipline*" in 1972)*
The requirements of the deliberative nursing process (nursing process discipline) are: (a) what the nurse says verbally or conveys nonverbally to the individual must match any or all of the items of her or his immediate reaction, (b) the nurse must clearly express it as self-designated, and (c) the nurse must ask correction or verification from that other person (Orlando, 1972).

Distress
Patients become distressed when they cannot, without help, cope with their needs (Orlando, 1961).

Evaluation of nurse activity
Because a nurse's activity is professional only when the nurse deliberatively achieves the purpose of helping the patient, the activity is

not the criterion by which it may be evaluated. The relevance and significance of an activity are determined by whether it helps the patient communicate his or her needs and how the need for help is being met (Orlando, 1961).

Immediate reaction
A person's perception through one of the five sense organs, the automatic thought stimulated by the perception, and the feeling the person experiences following the thought.

Improvement (also see Product)
The patient's immediate improvement is relative to what it was when the process started, and is concerned with increases in the patient's sense of well-being or a change for the better in his or her condition (Orlando, 1961).

Need
"Need is situationally defined as a requirement of the patient which, if supplied, relieves or diminishes his immediate distress or improves his immediate sense of adequacy or well-being" (Orlando, 1961, p. 5).

Nurse's practice
"Learning how to understand what is happening between herself and the patient is the central core of the nurse's practice and comprises the basic framework for the help she gives to patients" (Orlando, 1961, p. 4).

Nursing
"Nursing . . . is responsive to individuals who suffer or anticipate a sense of helplessness; it is focused on the process of care in an immediate experience; it is concerned with providing direct assistance to individuals in whatever setting they are found for the purpose of avoiding, relieving, diminishing or curing the individual's sense of helplessness" (Orlando, 1972, p. 12).

Nursing process
The elements of nursing process are the patient's behavior, the nurse's reaction, and the nursing action (Orlando, 1961).

Nursing process discipline (see "Deliberative nursing process"*)*

Nursing situation
Three basic elements make up a nursing situation: (a) the patient's behavior, (b) the nurse's reaction, and (c) the nursing actions designed for the patient's benefit (Orlando, 1961).

Nursing's purpose
"The purpose of nursing is to supply the help a patient requires for his needs to be met" (Orlando, 1961, p. 8).

Presenting behavior
"The presenting behavior of the patient, regardless of the form in which it appears, may represent a plea for help" (Orlando, 1961, p. 40).

Product
"The product of meeting the patient's immediate need for help is ... 'improvement' in the immediate verbal and nonverbal behavior of the patient" (Orlando, 1972, p. 21).

"The product of professional nursing must be formulated in terms of what professional nursing aims to accomplish, that is, the individual's restoration or improvement in the capacity to care for the self" (Orlando & Dugan, 1989, p. 79).

Professional function of nursing
"The function of professional nursing is ... conceptualized as finding out and meeting the patient's immediate needs for help" (Orlando, 1972, p. 20).

Situational conflict
At the start of any nurse-patient contact, an almost inevitable conflict occurs between an automatic activity and the patient's immediate need, which may be described as a *situational conflict* (Orlando, 1961).

References

Anderson, B. J., Mertz, H., & Leonard, R. C. (1965). Two experimental tests of a patient-centered admission process. *Nursing Research, 14*(2), 151-157.

Andrews, C. M. (1989). Ida Orlando's model of nursing practice. In J. J. Fitzpatrick & A. L. Whall (Eds.), *Conceptual models of nursing analysis and application* (2nd ed.) (Chap. 6). Norwalk, CT: Appleton & Lange.

Argyris, C., & Schön, D. (1978). *Organizational learning: A theory of action perspective.* Reading, MA: Addison-Wesley.

Barnum, B. J. S. (1990). *Nursing theory analysis, application, evaluation* (3rd ed.). Glenview, IL: Scott, Foresman/Little, Brown Education.

Barron, M. A. (1966). The effects varied nursing approaches have on patients' complaints of pain. *Nursing Research, 15*(1), 90-91.

Bochnak, M. A. (1963). The effect of an automatic and deliberative process of nursing activity on the relief of patients' pain: A clinical experiment. *Nursing Research, 12*(3), 191-192.

Bochnak, M. A., Rhymes, J. P., & Leonard, R. C. (1962). The comparison of two types of nursing activity on the relief of pain. In *Innovations in nurse-patient relationships: Automatic or reasoned nurse action* (Clinical Paper No. 6). New York: American Nurses' Association.

Burr, W. R., Hill, R., Nye, F. I., & Reiss, I. L. (Eds.). (1979). *Contemporary theories about the family.* New York: Free Press.

Cameron, J. (1962). The patient needs to be understood. In *Innovations in nurse-patient relationships: Automatic or reasoned nurse action* (Clinical Paper No. 19). New York: American Nurses' Association.

Cameron, J. (1963). An exploratory study of the verbal responses of the nurse-patient interactions. *Nursing Research, 12*(3), 192.

Clausen [Cameron], J. C. (1983). Clinical nursing research on the science and art of breastfeeding using a deliberative nursing care approach. *Western Journal of Nursing Research, 5*(3), 29.

Dewey, J. (1933). *How we think: A restatement of the relation of reflective thinking to the educative process.* Boston: D. C. Heath.

Dewey, J. (1938). *Logic: The theory of inquiry.* New York: Holt, Rinehart & Winston.

Dumas, R. G. (1963). Psychological preparation for surgery. *The American Journal of Nursing, 63*(8), 52-55.

Dumas, R. G., Anderson, B. J., & Leonard, R. C. (1965). The importance of the expressive function in preoperative preparation. In J. K. Skipper, Jr., & R. C. Leonard (Eds.), *Social interaction and patient care* (pp. 16-29). Philadelphia: J. B. Lippincott.

Dumas, R. G., & Johnson [Anderson], B. A. (1972). Research in nursing practice: A review of five clinical experiments. *International Journal of Nursing Studies, 9,* 137-149.

Dumas, R. G., & Leonard, R. C. (1963). The effect of nursing on the incidence of postoperative vomiting. *Nursing Research, 12*(1), 12-15.

Dye, M. C. (1963a). Clarifying patients' communication. *The American Journal of Nursing, 63*(8), 56-59.

Dye, M. C. (1963b). A descriptive study of conditions conducive to an effective process of nursing activity. *Nursing Research, 12*(3), 194.

Elder, R. G. (1963). What is the patient saying? *Nursing Forum, 2*(1), 25-37.

Elms, R. R. (1964). Effects of varied nursing approaches during hospital admission: An exploratory study. *Nursing Research, 13*(3), 266-268.

Elms, R. R., & Leonard, R. C. (1966). Effects of nursing approaches during admission. *Nursing Research, 15*(1), 39-48.

Faulkner, S. A. (1963). A descriptive study of needs communicated to the nurse by some mothers on a postpartum service. *Nursing Research, 4*(12), 260.

Fischelis, M. C. (1963). An exploratory study of labels nurses attach to patient behavior and their effect on nursing activities. *Nursing Research, 12*(3), 195.

Gilbert, R. (1940). *The public health nurse and her patient.* New York: Commonwealth Fund.

Gilbert, R. (1951). *The public health nurse and her patient* (2nd ed.). Cambridge, MA: Harvard University Press.

Gillis, Sister L. (1976). Sleeplessness: Can you help? *The Canadian Nurse, 72*(7), 32-34.

Gowan, N. I., & Morris, M. (1964). Nurses' responses to expressed patient needs. *Nursing Research, 13*(1), 68-71.

Haggerty, L. A. (1987). An analysis of senior nursing students' immediate responses to distressed patients. *Journal of Advanced Nursing, 12,* 451-461.

Harré, R. (1989). *The philosophies of science* (2nd ed.). Oxford and New York: Oxford University Press.

Hopkins, L. T. (1941). *Interaction: The democratic process.* Boston: D. C. Heath.

Hopkins, L. T. (1954). *The emerging self in school and home.* New York: Harper & Brothers.

Kilpatrick, W. H. (1925). *Foundations of method: Informal talks in teaching.* New York: Macmillan.

Kilpatrick, W. H. (1941). *Selfhood and civilization: A study of the self-other process.* New York: Columbia University, Teachers College.

Kim, H. S. (1983). *The nature of theoretical thinking in nursing.* Norwalk, CT: Appleton-Century-Crofts.

Kuhn, T. S. (1970). *The structure of scientific revolutions* (2nd ed.). Chicago: University of Chicago Press.

Leonard, M. K., & Crane, M. D. (1990). Ida Jean Orlando. In J. B. George (Ed.), *Nursing theories: The base for professional nursing practice* (3rd ed.) (Chap. 10). Norwalk, CT: Appleton & Lange.

Marriner-Tomey, A. (Ed.). (1989). *Nursing theorists and their work* (2nd ed.) (Chap. 19). St. Louis, MO: C. V. Mosby.

McManus, R. L. (1948). *The effect of experience on nursing achievement.* New York: Columbia University, Teachers College, Bureau of Publications.

Meleis, A. I. (1991). *Theoretical nursing development and progress* (2nd ed.). Philadelphia: J. B. Lippincott.

Mertz, H. (1963). A study of the process of the nurse's activity as it affects the blood pressure readings and pulse rate of patients admitted to the emergency room. *Nursing Research, 12*(3), 197-198.

Orlando, I. J. (1961). *The dynamic nurse-patient relationship, function, process and principles.* New York: G. P. Putnam.

Orlando, I. J. (1972). *The discipline and teaching of nursing process: An evaluative study.* New York: G. P. Putnam.

Orlando [Pelletier], I. J. (1983, October). *Comments on ANA's social policy statement of 1980.* Paper presented at Southeastern Massachusetts University, College of Nursing, Honor Society, South Dartmouth, MA.

Orlando, I. J. (1985, October). *Nursing in the 21st century: Alternate paths.* Paper presented at Oakland University, School of Nursing, Rochester, MI.

Orlando, I. J. (1987). Nursing in the 21st century: Alternate paths. *Journal of Advanced Nursing, 12,* 405-412.

Orlando, I. J., & Dugan, A. B. (1989). Independent and dependent paths: The fundamental issue for the nursing profession. *Nursing and Health Care, 10*(2), 77-80.

Pelletier, I. J. (1976, August). *The fundamental issue in professional nursing.* Paper presented at University of Tulsa, College of Nursing, Tulsa, OK.

Pelletier, I. O. (1967). The patient's predicament and nursing function. *Psychiatric Opinion, 4,* 25-29.

Pelletier, I. O. (1968, May 3). *Nursing process and the problem of evaluating its effectiveness.* Unpublished presentation. Academic Conference, McLean Hospital, Belmont, MA.

Pelletier, I. O. (1980). *Commentary on ANA draft report, The nature and scope of nursing practice characteristics of specialization: A social policy statement.* Unpublished manuscript.

Peplau, H. E. (1952). *Interpersonal relations in nursing: A conceptual frame of reference for psychodynamic nursing.* New York: G. P. Putnam.

Ponte, P. R. (1988). *The relationship among empathy and the use of Orlando's deliberative process by the primary nurse and the distress of the adult cancer patient.* Doctoral dissertation, Boston University, Boston.

Pride, L. F. (1968). An adrenal stress index as a criterion measure of nursing. *Nursing Research, 17*(4), 292-303.

Rhymes, J. (1964). A description of nurse-patient interaction in effective nursing activity. *Nursing Research, 13*(4), 365.

Schmieding, N. J. (1983). The analysis of Orlando's nursing theory based on Kuhn's theory of science. In P. Chinn (Ed.), *Advances in nursing theory development* (pp. 63-87). Rockville, MD: Aspen Systems.

Schmieding, N. J. (1986). Orlando's theory. In P. Winstead-Fry (Ed.), *Case studies in nursing theory*, pp. 1-36. New York: National League for Nursing.

Schmieding, N. J. (1987). Problematic situations in nursing: Analysis of Orlando's theory based on Dewey's theory of inquiry. *Journal of Advanced Nursing, 12*(4), 431-440.

Schmieding, N. J. (1988). Action process of nurse administrators to problematic situations based on Orlando's theory. *Journal of Advanced Nursing, 13*(1), 99-107.

Schmieding, N. J. (1990a). Do head nurses include staff nurses in problem solving? *Nursing Management, 21*(3), 58-60.

Schmieding, N. J. (1990b). A model for assessing nurse administrator's actions. *Western Journal of Nursing Research, 12*(3), 293-306.

Schmieding, N. J. (1992). Relationship between head nurse responses to staff nurses and staff nurse response to patients. *Western Journal of Nursing Research, 13*(6), 746-760.

Tarasuk [Bochnak], M. B., Rhymes, J., & Leonard, R. C. (1965). An experimental test of the importance of communication skills for effective nursing. In J. K. Skipper, Jr., & R. C. Leonard (Eds.), *Social interaction and patient care* (pp. 110-120). Philadelphia: J. B. Lippincott.

Thibaudeau, M., & Reidy, M. M. (1977). Nursing makes a difference: A comparative study of the health behavior of mothers in three primary care agencies. *International Journal of Nursing, 14*, 97-107.

Torres, G. (1990). The place of concepts and theories within nursing. In J. B. George (Ed.), *Nursing theories: The base for professional nursing practice* (3rd ed.) (Chap. 1). Norwalk, CT: Appleton & Lange.

Tryon, P. A. (1962). The effect of patient participation in decision making on the outcome of a nursing procedure. In *Nursing and the patients' motivation* (Clinical Paper No. 19). New York: American Nurses' Association.

Tryon, P. A. (1966). Use of comfort measures as support during labor. *Nursing Research, 15*(2), 109-118.

Tryon, P. A., & Leonard, R. C. (1964). The effect of patients' participation on the outcome of a nursing procedure. *Nursing Forum, 3*(2), 79-89.

Walker, L. O. (1992). Theory, practice, and research in perspective. In L. H. Nicoll (Ed.), *Perspectives on nursing theory* (2nd ed.) (Chap. 5). New York: J. B. Lippincott.

Wolfer, J., & Visintainer, M. A. (1975). Pediatric surgical patients' and parents' stress response and adjustment as a function of psychological preparation and stress point nursing care. *Nursing Research, 24*(4), 244-255.

Bibliography

References Related to Orlando's Work

Allen, M., Frasure-Smith, N., & Gottlieb, L. (1982). What makes a "good" nurse? *The Canadian Nurse, 78,* 42-45.

Bottorff, J. L., & D'Cruz, J. V. (1984). Towards inclusive notions of "patient" and "nurse." *Journal of Advanced Nursing, 9,* 549-553.

Chapman, J. S. (1969). *Effects of different nursing approaches upon psychological and physiological responses of patients.* Cleveland, OH: Case Western Reserve University, Frances Payne Bolton School of Nursing.

Dracup, K. A., & Breu, C. S. (1978). Using nursing research findings to meet the needs of grieving spouses. *Nursing Research, 27*(4), 212-216.

Eisler, J., Wolfer, J. A., & Diers, D. (1972). Relationship between need for social approval and postoperative recovery and welfare. *Nursing Research, 21*(5), 520-525.

Farrell, G. A. (1991). How accurately do nurses perceive patients' needs? A comparison of general and psychiatric settings. *Journal of Advanced Nursing, 16,* 1062-1070.

Forchuk, C. (1991). A comparison of the works of Peplau and Orlando. *Archives of Psychiatric Nursing, 5,* 38-45.

Haggerty, L. A. (1985). A theoretical model for developing students' communication skills. *Journal of Nursing Education, 24*(7), 296-298.

Hampe, S. O. (1975). Needs of grieving spouses in a hospital setting. *Nursing Research, 24*(2), 113.

Harrison, C. (1966). Deliberative nursing process versus automatic nurse action. *Nursing Clinics of North America, 1*(3), 387-397.

Kokuyama, T., & Schmieding, N. J. (in press). Responses staff nurses prefer compared with their perception of head nurse responses. *Japanese Journal of Nursing Administration.*

58   IDA JEAN ORLANDO

Kumata, M., & Goto, H. (1984). What I learned from Orlando—Individuality and determination in actual interaction with a patient. *Gekkan Nursing, 4*(4), 129-133.

Lego, S. (1975). The one-to-one nurse-patient relationship. In *Psychiatric nursing 1946 to 1974: A report on the state of the art—Completed by Florence L. Huey* (pp. 1-61). New York: American Journal of Nursing Company.

Mahaffy, P. P. (1965). The effects of hospitalization on children admitted for tonsillectomy and adenoidectomy. *Nursing Research, 14*(1), 12-19.

Marriner-Tomey, A., Mills, D. I., & Sauter, M. K. (1989). Ida Jean Orlando (Pelletier) nursing process theory. In A. Marriner-Tomey (Ed.), *Nursing theorists and their work* (2nd ed.) (Chap. 19). St. Louis, MO: C. V. Mosby.

Nelson, B. (1978). A practical application of nursing theory. *Nursing Clinics of North America, 13*(1), 157-169.

New England Board of Higher Education. (1977). *Mental health continuing education for associate degree nursing faculties: Project report* (NIH Training Grant #715 MH13182). Wellesley, MA: Author.

Peitchinis, J. A. (1972). Therapeutic effectiveness of counseling by nursing personnel. *Nursing Research, 21*(2), 138-148.

Perry, J. (1985). Has the discipline of nursing developed to the stage where nurses do "think nursing?" *Journal of Advanced Nursing, 10,* 31-37.

Phillips, S. J. (1988). *Clinical judgment of students in professional nursing programs: An inductive approach.* Unpublished doctoral dissertation, Case Western Reserve University, Cleveland, OH.

Powell, J. H. (1989). The reflective practitioner in nursing. *Journal of Advanced Nursing, 14,* 824-832.

Schmieding, N. J. (1970). The relationship of nursing to the process of chronicity. *Nursing Outlook, 18*(2), 58-62.

Schmieding, N. J. (1983). A description and analysis of the directive process used by directors of nursing, supervisors, and head nurses in problematic situations based on Orlando's theory of nursing experience. Doctoral dissertation, Boston University, Boston. (Microfilm No. 83-19936)

Schmieding, N. J. (1984). Putting Orlando's theory into practice. *American Journal of Nursing, 84*(6), 759-761.

Schmieding, N. J. (1987). Analyzing managerial responses in face-to-face contacts. *Journal of Advanced Nursing, 12*(3), 357-365.

Schmieding, N. J. (1987). Face-to-face contacts: Exploring their meaning. *Nursing Management, 12*(11), 82-86.

Schmieding, N. J. (1990). The analysis of the patient's immediate experience through the use of Orlando's theory. In *Proceedings of the first and second Rosemary Ellis scholars' retreat* (pp. 155-158). Cleveland, OH: Case Western Reserve University, Frances Payne Bolton School of Nursing.

Schmieding, N. J. (1990). Foreword. In I. J. Orlando, *The dynamic nurse-patient relationship: Function, process and principle* (pp. xvii-xix). New York: National League for Nursing.

Schmieding, N. J. (1990). An integrative nursing theoretical framework. *Journal of Advanced Nursing, 15*(4), 463-467.

Schmieding, N. J. (1993). Empowerment through context, structure, and process. *Journal of Professional Nursing, 9*(4), 239-245.

Schmieding, N. J. (1993). Successful superior-subordinate relationships require mutual management. *Health Care Supervisor, 11*(4), 52-63.

Silva, M. C. (1979). Effects of orientation information on spouses' anxieties and attitudes toward hospitalization and surgery. *Research in Nursing and Health, 2,* 127-136.

Skipper, J. K., Jr., Leonard, R. C., & Rhymes, J. (1968). Child hospitalization and social interaction: An experimental study of mothers' feelings of stress, adaptation and satisfaction. *Medical Care, 6*(6), 496-506.

Wallston, K. A., Cohen, B. D., Wallston, B. S., Smith, R. A., & DeVellis, B. M. (1978). Increasing nurses' person-centeredness. *Nursing Research, 27*(3), 156-159.

Wiedenbach, E. (1958). *Family-centered maternity nursing.* New York: G. P. Putnam.

Williamson, Y. M. (1978). Methodologic dilemmas in tapping the concept of patient needs. *Nursing Research, 27*(3), 172-177.

Wooldridge, P. J., Leonard, R. C., & Skipper, J. K., Jr. (1978). *Methods of clinical experimentation to improve patient care.* St. Louis, MO: C. V. Mosby.

About the Author

Norma Jean Schmieding, Ed.D., R.N., is Professor of Nursing at the University of Rhode Island College of Nursing. She is a diploma graduate of Lincoln General Hospital School of Nursing, Lincoln, Nebraska, and has a B.S. from Nebraska Wesleyan University, also in Lincoln. Her master's in nursing administration was obtained at Boston University, where she also received her doctorate in 1983. Her career has been divided between nursing service and nursing education. In the early 1970s as Director of Nursing Service at Boston City Hospital she implemented Orlando's theory. She is an expert on Orlando's theory and has used it extensively in nursing service and research. Her publications include those on theoretical and concept analyses, research, and application to nursing service.